FOR THE DURATION

Though less catastrophic than AIDS, herpes is still a major health problem—and one that won't go away, as herpes infections last for life, and must be managed, not cured. Anti-herpes drugs have been varyingly effective, and in any case are often expensive and carry objectionable side effects. Dr. Jan de Vries offers the good news of a nature-derived remedy that has shown effectiveness against herpes, as well as against other unpleasant viral conditions. Learn what part Melissa extract may play in your own health program.

ABOUT THE AUTHOR

Jan de Vries, born in Holland, took a degree in pharmacy, but soon became an expert in alternative medicine. He has worked closely with Alfred Vogel, the famous "Swiss Nature Doctor," for more than 35 years, and now practices homeopathy, osteopathy, naturopathy and acupuncture in clinics he has established in the U.K. and Holland. He appears regularly on BBC Radio, promoting his philosophy of "Health for Everyone—naturally."

Melissa Extract: The Natural Herbal Remedy for Herpes

Safe treatment for one of the most widespread and insidious diseases

Jan de Vries

Keats Publishing, Inc. New Canaan, Connecticut

CONTENTS

If you are one of the millions of people who are plagued by cold sores or genital herpes—both offspring of the conniving herpes family of viruses—you have probably considered escaping to a deserted island until the scourge has passed. Even the unsightly cold sores on your lip, although not life-threatening, are nevertheless in plain view for all to see.

Genital herpes is even more embarrassing. Although only visible during intimate contact, the repulsive lesions are enough to put your sex life on hold indefinitely. Needless to say, the herpes family is as difficult to shake as a pesky salesman. And like unfriendly relatives, they remain with you for life.

Because health care costs continue to skyrocket, and because prescribed drugs are expensive and often leave debilitating side effects, more and more people are turning to alternative therapies. These natural remedies are usually less expensive than prescribed drugs, and the side effects, if any, are minimal.[1]

In the book, *New Choices in Natural Healing*, Varro E. Tyler, Ph.D., professor of pharmacognosy at Purdue University, is quoted as saying that Europeans depend on *Melissa officinalis* (lemon balm) to treat cold sores caused by the herpes simplex virus. That's because the herb has antibacterial and antiviral properties.[2]

A melissa cream now available in American health food stores is effective in the treatment of genital herpes. This cream employs the therapeutically proven 70:1 extract; that is, 70 grams of the herb are treated by a special process to produce 1 gram of extract.

This process permits enrichment of the active antiviral principles of melissa, as assured by tests, and the elimination of inactive components, so that the resulting fraction, or chemical complex, is far more bioactive than the original plant. The historical material I go into later on deals with the plant, but most of the scientific studies I cite employed the 70:1 extract, which is now really the preferred form.

Later we shall see how the extract of this powerful herb deals with cold sores and genial herpes, as well as many other illnesses and health problems.

INTRODUCTION

Before the AIDS epidemic hogged the headlines, genital herpes was a sexual scourge that was constantly in the news. Genital herpes is still the most common venereal disease in the United States, with roughly 20 million Americans infected. According to Robert M. Giller, M.D., there are an estimated 500,000 new cases annually.[1]

Sexually transmitted diseases pose a major health problem, reports the *ABC's of the Human Body*. In the United States and Canada, there are four particularly troublesome sexually related diseases, not including AIDS. Chlamydia is a major cause of sterility in women. Gonorrhea, the second most common, is somewhat easy to cure in its initial stages, but it is often difficult to detect. Genital herpes, although not considered life-threatening, is a recurrent illness and is so far uncurable. The fourth, syphilis, is the least prevalent sexually transmitted disease, but it is the most dangerous. Less threatening sexual diseases include chancroid, a condition that results in soft ulcers; venereal warts, which are caused by a virus that attacks mostly women; and trichomoniasis, a form of vaginitis that usually does not cause symptoms in males.[2]

According to the September 1995 issue of *Longevity*, when herpes initially occurs, the length of time it hangs around seems to predict future flare-ups. In other words, the longer the first attack, the more often herpes is likely to reappear. Men are more likely to be involved with that scenario.

"A study by researchers at the University of Washington in Seattle found that, of 457 patients with genital herpes, those whose first infection lasted longer than 35 days had twice as many recurrences as those with shorter first-time infections," stated Carol Potera. "Just 8 percent of men escaped recurrences, compared to 26 percent of women. And 26 percent of men had 10 more recurrences over the course of the year—the overall average was four. The higher number of flare-ups in men helps explain why more women are infected with genital herpes by men than men are infected by women." Lawrence Corey, M.D., professor of medicine at the University of Washington, added that "Abstaining from sex during recurrences prevents transmission."[3]

The other side of the coin are cold sores (fever blisters), which are caused by the herpes simplex virus. Although an infection of the mouth is rather common and does not necessarily pose a serious health risk, a danger arises if, during the initial infection, you touch the ulcers and then your eyes, which could result in a herpetic corneal ulcer. (The cornea, a transparent covering at the very front of the eye, is most susceptible to injury and infection.) Though painful, infections caused by herpes simplex virus are invisible to the naked eye.[4]

Many viruses have evolved mechanisms to avoid detection by the host immune system, reports a 1995 article in *Nature*. It's rather complicated, but the herpes simplex virus releases an immediate early protein, ICP47, which blocks presentation of viral peptides to MHC class 1-restricted cells. The researchers show that ICP47 binds to antigen processing and prevents peptides from moving into the connective tissue fiber between cells.[5]

Recent research shows herpes viruses may cause or somehow be linked to other diseases such as chronic fatigue syndrome and hardening of the arteries. In a 1992 article in the *Sacramento Bee*, for instance, Richard A. Knox reported that a recent in-depth study of chronic fatigue syndrome patients showed that a majority had brain damage and evidence of active viral infection by herpes virus 6, a newly discovered strain. Seventy percent of the chronic fatigue patients had evidence of active infection by human herpes virus 6, compared with 20 percent of the controls infected with the virus. It was found that patients with this syndrome had evidence of immune function abnormalities that suggested an active viral infection. It is not known whether brain damage occurs because of herpes virus 6 or inflammatory chemicals.[6]

In a general review article in the 1992 *Israel Journal of Medical Sciences*, Joseph Melnick and Arni Schattner discussed intriguing data supporting the possibility that early arterial infection by herpes viruses, especially cytomegalovirus, may initiate hardening of the arteries. They came to their conclusions after evaluating (1) herpes virus-induced atherosclerosis in birds, (2) the combination of data from sensitive assays which detect cytomegalovirus-encoded proteins in arterial tissue of patients, (3) the important recent link between atherosclerosis and transplanted hearts and posttransplantation cytomegalovirus infection, and (4) the discovery of the biological characteristics of the arterial cell infection by cytomegalovirus.[7] Further research is needed to substantiate the causal relationship between herpes viruses and hardening of the arteries. Maybe someday it will be shown that herpes viruses have a far more profound role in causing illnesses than has been previously thought.

LEARNING MORE ABOUT YOUR SKIN

Your skin, one of the largest organs in your body, is a supple, elastic tissue that conserves moisture and heat. It also provides useful information about your surroundings.

Buried in your skin are millions of tiny nerve endings called receptors, which sense touch, pressure, heat, cold and pain. Also embedded in your skin are numerous minute glands. As an example, there are sebaceous glands, which produce a waxy substance that helps keep your skin surface supple and perhaps prevents it from drying out. And there are sweat glands, which produce a watery liquid (perspiration) to cool you when you are too hot—it's the evaporation of the sweat from your skin that cools you. To assist with temperature regulation, the small blood vessels in your skin expand in hot weather to lose heat, giving you a flushed appearance. The same vessels constrict in cold weather to conserve heat.

The skin is composed of two layers. The thin surface layer is called the epidermis; below that is the thicker layer, the dermis. The epidermis is an active layer of cells, in that the cells at its base are constantly dividing to produce new cells, which gradually die as they fill up with a hard substance called keratin. As the cells die, they move to the surface of the skin to be shed or worn away by rubbing from your clothes, washing or handling things.

"The continuous production of cells at the base of the epidermis keeps up with continuous loss of cells from its surface," explains *The American Medical Association Family Medical Guide.* "It takes an average of one month for any single epidermal cell to complete the journey from base to surface. On parts of the body where pressure and friction are greatest, the epidermis is thicker and the journey takes longer. A number of skin problems are caused by a fault in the constant turnover of skin cells."

The AMA guide continues, "Because your skin, hair and nails are on the outside of your body, you quickly notice any change in their appearance. In fact, most of the problems in these areas relate mainly to changes in appearance. There may be symptoms such as itching, swelling, or, occasionally, pain. Diseases of the skin, hair and nails can be irritating and uncomfortable. They can also be embarrassing because of their appearance."[1]

In their informative book, *Do-It-Yourself Medical Testing*, Cathey Pinckney and Edward R. Pinckney, M.D., discuss the many ways you can determine whether or not you have a skin problem. Although researchers describe skin changes in a variety of ways, the following three characteristics are usually involved:

COLOR

The presence or absence of pigment—which usually does not include generalized redness—should be noted.

PHYSICAL STRUCTURE

Some abnormalities include macules, which are lesions, usually colored, that are not elevated above the skin's surface (they cannot be felt as bumps when touched); papules, which are raised above the skin's surface, somewhat like a mosquito bite, can be felt; skin plaques, which are large papules; vesicles or bullae, which are blisterlike lesions containing fluid (when infected, they are called pustules).

BLANCHABILITY

You should observe whether or not the skin's color disappears when pressure is applied by a fingertip.

Skin lesions should be distinguished from eczema, an inflammation of the skin, and from hives, an allergic reaction in which red, pink or sometimes pale swollen patches arise suddenly but are rarely permanent. Drugs can also cause a variety of skin conditions, often prompted or promoted by sunlight. Antibiotics, aspirin and aspirin-like medications, birth control pills, food colorings, diuretics and even some vitamins commonly cause skin rashes.

Diet can also be related to skin lesions. As an example, several reports show that a diet high in polyunsaturated fats is associated with several different cancers—malignant melanoma in particular. Should one or two reddish pimples erupt on your nose or face one morning, try to recall whether you have eaten any beef in the last day or two. The female hormones used to fatten cattle can cause an acne-like reaction in susceptible people.

The sudden appearance of brown pigmentation, especially on exposed surfaces, can be the first indication of an adrenal gland disorder (Addison's disease); it can also come from anemia, cancer and other connective tissue conditions. Some women taking birth control pills also develop areas of brown pigmentation that appear most often over the cheekbones and around the nipples.

"Tiny clusters or blisters appearing around the mouth (cold sores) are usually caused by a herpes virus," say the Pinckneys. "It is believed that once the virus establishes itself in the body—usually in the nerves—it remains for a lifetime and can be reactivated by upper respiratory infections, sunlight, stress and steroid (cortisone) drugs. The same form of herpes virus or a different, second, form can also cause blisters to appear on and around the genitalia."[2]

Herpes-like blisters, especially on or around the genitalia, warrant medical attention to ascertain the diagnosis—both to protect others from catching the disease and because, if the condition is found in a pregnant woman, it can cause brain damage and death in newborns. And herpes-type lesions have frequently been associated with cancer of the cervix and lymph cell cancers such as leukemia.

HOW HERPES ENTERS A CELL

Although some researchers remain skeptical, a clue as to how the herpes virus enters a cell was announced in *Science* in 1990 by David P. Hajjar, M.D., a professor of biochemistry and pathology at Cornell Medical Center in New York. In related studies, other scientists suggested that there is evidence that the virus is linked to atherosclerosis or hardening of the arteries, reported Natalie Angier in *The New York Times*.[1]

Hajjar and his colleagues determined that the herpes simplex 1 virus infiltrates its target by piggybacking on a vital hormonelike protein that cells need to survive. They have yet to find out whether or not herpes simplex 2 virus, which causes genital herpes, infects cells in a similar way.

In their experiments, Hajjar and his co-workers showed that the herpes virus invades cells through a type of protein known as a receptor on the outer membrane of many cells. The usual role of the receptor is to grasp molecules of a protein called fibroblast growth factor, which float in the bloodstream, and yank them into the cell. Once inside the cell, the growth factor stimulates cell division or performs a similar growth-related task.

"The Cornell work suggests that the herpes virus latches onto fibroblast growth factor and is pulled into the cell coincidentally by the receptor," wrote Angier. "In one experiment, the scientists demonstrated that when they blocked the receptor with a decoy compound, the herpes virus had great difficulty infecting the cells. Hajjar said that 70 percent of the viruses could not enter the cells. And he believes the rest slipped inside either accidentally, or by another, minor pathway."

The New York scientists are now working to develop a drug that mimics the shape of the growth factor, in the hope that it will interfere with a herpes infection by soaking up viruses before they have a chance to attach themselves to the genuine growth proteins in the body. However, unlike the natural growth factors, the mock drug will apparently not be able to link up with the cell receptor; therefore, the virus will be prevented from being taken into cells.

Hajjar also believes that such a drug could help prevent atherosclerosis. He bases that on studies showing that herpes infection caused hardened arteries in animals. Scientists have also found traces of genetic material and proteins from the herpes virus in plaques clogging the arteries of people with atherosclerosis. In addition, researchers reported detecting cytomegalovirus, a relative of herpes simplex 1, in human arterial plaques.

Hajjar theorizes that the herpes virus may cause hardening of the arteries by infecting the cells of the arterial walls, altering how cholesterol is metabolized. His research suggests that the virus suppresses the activity of enzymes that normally break down stored cholesterol in the cell. That inhibition possibly leads to the accumulation of cholesterol plaques. In time, plaques can cut off the flow of blood to the heart, contributing to a heart attack.

"Herpes is one of the most widespread viruses in the United States, and now we know how it gets into cells," Hajjar was quoted as saying. "If we can nail down the connection between herpes and atherosclerosis, then this discovery will have major, major ramifications."

COLD SORES AND FEVER BLISTERS

Cold sores, also called fever blisters, are caused by the herpes simplex 1 virus. They generally form on the outside of the mouth, affecting the lips and the skin around the lips. The minute blisters, which are highly contagious, are filled with clear fluid and form on a patch of red and slightly raised skin. The blisters occur in small clusters; however, several groups can merge to cover an area of half an inch or more.

Before the blisters surface, there is often a feeling of fullness, burning or itching. After they erupt, the blisters become larger, burst and begin to dry out. The sores usually heal within two or three weeks, seldom leaving a scar. While in the latent stage between recurrences, the virus is not transmissible. Of primary concern when the herpes simplex 1 virus is active is that it may be transmitted to the eye, where it can ulcerate the cornea and cause blindness.

"About three-quarters of the population is infected by herpes simplex 1 for the first time in early childhood," reports *The Physicians' Manual for Patients.* "The incidence is particularly high among people living in crowded conditions and among those in the lower socioeconomic brackets. This primary infection often goes unnoticed because the blisters are so small. Sometimes, however, there is also loss of appetite, fever and considerable ulceration in the mouth. If the primary infection occurs in late childhood or the teen-age years, the virus may invade the bloodstream and cause severe systemic (bodywide) illness. In adults, in very rare cases, a primary systemic infection of herpes simplex 1 is fatal."[1]

After the initial infection, whether a mild or severe case,

antibodies to the virus develop in the bloodstream. Although the antibodies do not prevent a recurrence of the infection, they do make subsequent attacks less severe. The virus then lies dormant, apparently in the skin or in the nerve ganglia near the original site of the infection, often for years, until something triggers another eruption. The recurrence may be due to overexposure to sunlight, certain foods and drugs or physical or emotional stress. As an example, some febrile diseases, such as pneumonia, seem to stimulate a recurrence of cold sores.

Student nurses have a high incidence of cold sores, especially during times of "unhappiness," as measured by the Clyde Mood Scale, reported Eberhard Kronhausen, Ed.D., et al. in *Formula for Life*. "Examination anxiety can predispose students to a variety of infectious diseases," the authors said. "Researchers have studied a large group of West Point cadets over a four-year period with an eye to the relationship between academic stress and susceptibility to infectious mononucleosis (caused by the Epstein-Barr virus). Of the new cadets, 20 percent became infected each year and 25 percent actually developed the disease. The researchers were even able to predict a cadet's susceptibility to mononucleosis by tracking his reactions to the high academic demands and his performance on quizzes and examinations."[2]

The authors quoted studies that show that the increase in such infections is in direct proportion to the degree of examination anxiety reported by the students. The findings confirm similar studies on the link between academic stress and other infectious diseases. In one study, medical students were found to be most susceptible to the herpes viruses during periods of peak stress, especially those students who also had feelings of acute loneliness.

Since oral herpes is so contagious, kissing and other direct skin contact should be avoided. Sharing of eating utensils, lipsticks and the like should also be discouraged.[3]

GENITAL HERPES

Genital herpes, which is generally acquired by sexual intercourse with an infected person, is caused by either one of two closely related viruses, namely, herpes simplex 1 (HSV1) or herpes simplex 2 (HSV2). HSV2 is the most common cause of genital herpes and is found in 80 to 90 percent of initial infections and 95 percent of recurrent infections.

The incidence of infection is about 80 percent among prostitutes, 20 to 40 percent in lower socioeconomic groups, 10 percent in higher socioeconomic groups and only about 3 percent in celibate women. A person who is infected is most infectious when active skin lesions are present, but the virus can be found in the semen of 2 percent of infected men and in the cervical secretions of 4 percent of infected women, even when there are no apparent signs of the disease. And the infection can be transmitted to newborns as they pass through an infected birth canal.

HSV1 and HSV2 are members of the herpes virus family, which also includes the Epstein-Barr virus (the cause of infectious mononucleosis), the varicella-zoster virus (the cause of chickenpox and shingles) and cytomegalovirus (the cause of infections among newborns and patients with organ transplants).

The herpes virus consists of a core of deoxyribonucleic acid (DNA) surrounded by a protein coat that is covered by a membrane of lipid produced by the infected cell. Like other viruses, herpes can survive and multiply only inside a living cell, but in the process of multiplying they destroy the host cell. However, unlike most other viruses, herpes viruses can lie dormant in infected cells for long periods without harming the host cell. When triggered by a number of known and unknown factors, the virus becomes activated. Only then does it multiply and destroy the host cell, releasing a new infectious virus.

Genital herpes initially infects the skin, then travels up the sensory nerves from the skin to nerve cells of the sacral ganglia, near the spinal cord, where the virus becomes latent. Months or years later, the virus becomes activated, traveling down the nerves to the genital skin, causing a recurrent infection, even if no new exposure to an infection has occurred. The intermittent infection may or may not result in overt symptoms. Those with recurrent infections form a reservoir that allows herpes infections to persist.

The initial sign of infection is an itchy, painful red bump (papule), which appears two to eight days after intercourse. During the next several days, the papule turns into a 1- to 3-mm blister (vesicle), filled with clear fluid. For about ten days after the infection begins, the patient may feel ill, with fever, muscle aches, swelling of the lymph nodes in the groin, as well as pain while urinating. As the white blood cells attack the infection, the vesicle fluid turns cloudy and the vesicle ruptures, creating a small ulcer. The fluid released from the vesicles contains millions of viral particles that spread the infection to surrounding areas. The ulcers form a crust, or scab, eventually healing about four weeks after the infection began.

Although the genital skin is the most obvious site of the infection, the cervix (the neck of the uterus) is often involved when the infection begins in a woman. The infection can also affect the inner thighs, the buttocks and the breasts. If a severe headache begins, this may signify meningitis or an infection of the membranes around the brain. But recovery from this complication is generally complete.

The most difficult aspect of genital herpes is the recurrence of the infection, without any reinfection. A wide range of factors may prompt recurrence, including menstruation, stress and local trauma, and frequency of recurrence varies widely. One-half of all infected people have a recurrence within two to three months; 80 percent have a recurrence within six months.

A recurrent attack of genital herpes is generally less prolonged and severe than the first episode. A recurrence generally consists of pain and burning at the site of the infection, followed by the usual papule and vesicle and then healing within 10 to 14 days. However, recurrences may not produce any symptoms, and the patient may be unaware that he or she is infected.

A number of human cancers are associated with the herpes viruses. As an example, the Epstein-Barr virus has been associated with Burkitt's lymphoma (a cancer of lymph nodes discovered by Denis P. Burkitt, M.D., the English physician who later became famous for promoting bran and fiber in the diet) and nasopharyngeal carcinoma. Women with cervical cancer often shows signs of a previous herpes simplex virus (HSV) infection.

Genital herpes has been linked to cancer of the vulva, an aggressive tumor that can be treated only with extensive and disfiguring surgery, according to Bernadine Healy, M.D., in *A New Prescription for Women's Health*. However, most often, herpes is a source of pain and disfigurement and a reminder of some questionable past sexual encounters.[1]

Young women with HSV infections are said to develop premalignant changes of the cervix more frequently than women who have never had a herpes infection. And sensitive tests have revealed the presence of HSV proteins and DNA in cervical cancer cells. In lab tests, normal cervical cells assume some of the characteristics of cancer cells when infected with herpes simplex. HSV infection has also been noted in women with skin cancers in the genital area.

An infected woman can transmit HSV to her baby during childbirth if she has the active virus at the time of delivery. However, despite the frequency of HSV infections, only about 1 in 4,000 babies is infected. Because the infection often involves the brain, causing seizures and coma, the mortality rate is high (60 percent), with half the survivors having permanent damage. Fortunately, if active HSV infection is discovered before delivery, infection of the baby may be prevented by performing a Cesarean section.

Sexual practices involving oral-genital contact may be responsible for some crossover infections, while other crossover infections may be the result of self-infection through hand-genital-mouth contact. In males, the common sites of infection include the foreskin, the glans and the shaft of the penis. In females, the blister may occur on the labia, the clitoris, the opening of the vagina or occasionally on the cervix. Within a few days, the blisters rupture and merge to form large areas of denuded tissue surrounded by swollen inflamed skin.

Infections such as herpes and hepatitis have a proven link to standards of hygiene, reports Kenneth Seaton in the October 1991 issue of *High Tech Hygiene*. For example, sexual contact in humans often involves the areas of the fingertips and nails. And sexual secretions can contaminate the fingernails while removing a condom.[2] AIDS patients often die from secondary infections such as fungi, bacteria and viruses that can be spread by the fingernails and/or nails.

Seaton believes that personal hygiene, especially in the fingernail area and the surrounding skin, before and after sexual contact, is an effective way of preventing sexually transmitted diseases. He notes that there seems to be a low incidence of AIDS and sexually transmitted diseases in communities where ritualistic cleansing is practiced before and after sex, such as in the traditions of Jewish and Moslem women.

According to Rick A. Barbarash, Pharm.D., et al., in the Summer 1994 issue of the *Journal of the Advancement of Medicine*, the persistence of genital herpes was positively correlated with global levels of psychosocial distress as well as depression, somatoform symptoms, paranoid ideation and thought disorder.[3]

THE CHICKEN POX CONNECTION

Chicken pox is a somewhat mild infectious disease caused by the herpes zoster virus, sometimes referred to as *varicella zoster*. This is the same virus that, following years of dormancy, may cause shingles in adults. The virus usually affects only the skin and the lining of the mouth and throat. According to *The American Medical Association Family Medical Guide*, after it gets into the body, there is an incubation period of between 7 and 21 days.[1]

The name "chicken pox" is thought to come from the Latin word *cicer*, which means chickpea. The virus that causes chicken pox spreads so rapidly that most people have the disease by the time they are 15 years old. A person almost never has chicken pox twice. "The virus is spread by direct contact with infected persons or articles freshly soiled by the fluid from their blisters, or by airborne droplets expelled from their noses and throats when they cough or sneeze," reported *The People's Medical Manual*. "A person can pass on the disease for about a week or 10 days, possibly beginning one day before the rash appears and continuing until no new spots develop. The dry scabs are not infectious." A susceptible person will break out with chicken pox two or three weeks after being exposed. A child may also contract chicken pox from exposure to a person with shingles, which is caused by the same virus.[2]

"Although herpes viruses cause a wide variety of illnesses and have been studied extensively for the last few decades, they remain a medical enigma," stated *The Physicians' Manual for Patients*. "Once they invade the body, herpes viruses remain for life, although they may be dormant most of the time. Some, such as the varicella-zoster strain, may have different manifestations. This variety causes chicken pox in children, after which the virus remains in the nervous system. In most people, the virus never again becomes active, but for unknown reasons, in others it may erupt into painful attacks of herpes zoster (shingles). Similarly, herpes simplex also goes through recurring cycles of infectious activity and dormancy."[3]

WHERE SHINGLES FITS IN

As mentioned earlier, shingles (herpes zoster) is a painful viral infection which affects the nerve endings of the skin. Its name is derived from the Latin word *cingulum*, meaning belt or girdle, since the lesions tend to form around the belt area of the body.

"Shingles is the result of infection by the herpes zoster virus, the same virus that causes chicken pox," reported *The American Medical Association Family Medical Guide.* "During an attack of chicken pox the virus may find its way to the root of a nerve in the brain or spinal cord. It lies dormant there, often for many years, until it is reactivated. Then the virus multiplies and produces intense, knife-like pain in the nerve where it has lodged. It also causes a rash in the form of groups of blisters that appear on the skin that lies above the nerve. It is not known what reactivates the dormant herpes zoster virus."[1]

Shingles develops only in people who have had chicken pox. The reappearance of the virus can be triggered by an injury, emotional stress, certain drugs, exposure to cold and other factors, according to *The People's Medical Manual.* Shingles attacks are also rather common in cancer patients and others debilitated by severe illness and in people who have weakened immunological defenses. You cannot catch shingles from a person undergoing an attack, but if you come in direct contact with a shingles rash, you may come down with chicken pox if you've never had it.[2]

Most often seen in people over 60 years old, shingles can appear almost anywhere on the body, but it generally begins at the midline, or spine, and radiates around to the side or front of one side of the body, reported Michael Oxman, M.D., professor of medicine at the University of California at San Diego School of Medicine and chief of the infectious disease section at the Veterans Administration Medical Center in La Jolla, California.

"For the first half of our lives, we are repeatedly exposed to chicken pox," Oxman explained. "These repeated exposures serve to boost our immune system and keep the herpes virus in check. But as we age, we receive fewer and fewer exposures and our immune system seems to be less active. Therefore, when our immune system declines below a certain level, the virus can erupt as shingles. "This virus is smart enough to know that if it doesn't do much harm to its host, it will survive. It leads a quiet, benign life until conditions are right for it to emerge, such as age, exposure and the immune system."[3]

In healthy seniors, a bout with shingles is generally unpleasant, but in people whose immune systems are suppressed, including transplant patients or patients with Hodgkin's disease or AIDS, the situation is far more serious. In immunosuppressed patients, the incidence rate is 20 to 100 times higher than normal, and the outcome is more severe. The virus can produce pneumonia, liver disease or a number of serious complications that can be fatal.

WHAT HERPES TESTS ARE AVAILABLE

As we know, herpes simplex 1 virus causes oral cold sores and fever blisters, while herpes simplex 2 usually causes sores on and around the penis and vagina. To test for these conditions, scrapings from a suspect sore are examined under a microscope and/or cultured to determine whether it is caused by herpes. However, if there has been known exposure to a sexual partner with herpes, and the signs and symptoms are characteristic of herpes, testing is probably not necessary. But if it is not clear from the patient's history and symptoms whether they have herpes, these tests may provide an answer. Because a vaginal herpes infection can be transferred from the mother to the baby as it passes through the birth canal, any pregnant woman with herpes should have regular cultures during the last months of pregnancy. If herpes is active at the time of birth, a cesarean delivery is necessary to protect the baby.

Because of a suspected link between herpes and cervical cancer, women with recurrent herpes should have a Pap test every 6 to 12 months. [Named after Dr. George Papanicolaou (1883–1962), an American anatomist who developed the test, it involves a microscopic examination of cells taken as a smear (Pap smear) from a woman's cervix. It is used to detect uterine cancer in its early, treatable stage.]

There are two tests for herpes, neither of which requires any special preparation and no risks are involved:

Tzanck Test

Named after Arnault Tzanck (1886–1954), a Russian dermatologist, this test involves scraping the sore with a scalpel, and then the scrapings are spread on a slide and stained. A doctor examines the slide under a microscope, looking for giant cells and inclusion bodies that are characteristic of a herpes infection. Since the test is made during an office visit, results are available immediately. If no giant cells or inclusion bodies are found, the test is termed negative. However, there is a high rate of false-negative results (the test is negative though you really do have herpes).

Herpes Virus Culture

Scrapings and/or fluid from the lesions are collected on a cotton swab and sent to a laboratory that performs viral cultures. Results are usually available within 7 to 10 days. Although the culture is considerably more accurate than the Tzanck smear, it may also produce false-negative results if it is not done when the sores are fresh and active. If no herpes is found in the culture, the test is termed negative. If the virus is found, the test is positive.

"Sixty percent of us have some immunity to herpes viruses and are, therefore, extremely unlikely to get the disease," reported David S. Sobel, M.D., and Tom Ferguson, M.D., in *The People's Book of Medical Tests.* "While there is no cure for herpes, those with active outbreaks may find some relief with some recent medications. Fortunately, it appears that the disease is only contagious when active genital sores are present."[1]

VIROGEN HERPES SLIDE TEST

In 1985, Wampole Laboratories announced the availability of the Virogen Herpes Slide Test, which is said to produce results in as little as 30 minutes in a physician's office. "The importance of such a rapid and reliable Herpes test to both the medical and lay communities cannot be overemphasized," the company said. "Herpes simplex virus is widespread among the human population, and it is the cause of more eye and urogenital infections than any other virus. It is particularly important to diagnose patients who would be at risk of recurrence during pregnancy, because neonatal herpes infections carry a 50 to 70 percent risk of neonatal death."[2]

The test requires the pipetting of swab/culture media samples into separate rings of a disposable slide. A "specimen buffer/absorbent" is added and mixed for five minutes, followed by reagent and control latexes to the appropriate rings. After 25 minutes of additional rotation, a positive diagnosis is made from observing the level of graininess (agglutination) which develops in the various rings. If no agglutination is observed, the sample is then sent for cell culture confirmation.

ARE ALLERGIES INVOLVED?

In *Herpes Handbook*, Thomas R. Klosinski, D.C. reported that one of his patients broke out in herpes simplex lesions each time she drank red wine. A second patient had a herpes attack when he drank alcohol, and a third patient said that coffee brought on a herpes attack. Almost everyone has allergies to something, and allergies can often trigger a herpes attack.

"Things that can trigger an attack can be classified as being allergic, reactive or toxic to us," said Klosinski. "The difference is that while we may not be completely allergic to something, we could be reactive to it, or the substance may be toxic or poisonous to our system. What is bad for one person may be all right for someone else. We have to find out what our individual 'weaknesses' are in order to reduce herpes attacks and to avoid them whenever possible. This helps us to get in touch with our body and it is a good learning process in the long run."[1]

Klosinski has narrowed the list of foods and beverages that may trigger a herpes attack. They include:

- Foods that you crave. Cravings are a sign that you may be allergic to these foods or substances, since allergies and addiction go hand in hand. Some of the common cravings are fats, salt, dairy products, sugar, coffee, tea—you fill in your own cravings.
- Foods you consume a lot of. The more you consume a specific item, the greater your chances are of developing an allergy to it.
- Foods, beverages, drugs that precede a herpes attack. Keep a diary of anything consumed beginning with the first of the month. Note especially anything consumed or that you came in contact with 2 to 24 hours prior to the attack. This will enable you to avoid these substances in the future.
- Substances that make you sleepy or cause a headache. An early sign of an allergic reaction is tiredness, fatigue and irritability.
- Anything that raises your pulse. The following do-it-yourself allergy test can save you hundreds of dollars in doctors' visits. Make a suspect list of all the questionable foods, beverages, tobacco or drugs you want to test. You can find your pulse by pressing next to your Adam's apple or on the thumb side of your wrist.

  1. Take your pulse for a minute before consuming a questionable substance. Count the beats using a watch and write down the number.

2. Take your pulse 30 minutes after you have consumed these items. If your pulse goes up more than eight beats per minute, you probably have a reaction to something you ate, drank, smoked or came in contact with.
3. Keep a diary and record what you have ingested, your pulse rate and any symptoms you may have noticed—tiredness, heart palpitations, headache and so on.
4. Using the pulse test, isolate items one at a time from your suspect list. As an example, if your pulse went up after eating bread or wheat products, eat a piece of bread and nothing else. Check your pulse 15 to 30 minutes later to see if it is higher. If it is not, check the next item on your suspect list and so forth.

According to Klosinski, the most common allergens are:

Nightshade family (tobacco, peppers, potatoes, tomatoes)
Dairy products and beef
Gluten, a protein found in wheat, rye, oats and barley
Citrus fruits
Alcohol
Coffee and tea
Yeasts
Nitrates and nitrites found in processed meats
Eggs
Sugar
Monosodium glutamate (MSG)
Chocolate
Shellfish
Marijuana and other drugs

Klosinski notes that the rotation diet is beneficial for highly allergic people. This is how it works:

1. Keep a diary of everything you eat.
2. Do not eat the same things for four to five days. After three to four months, you may be able to reintroduce the things you were formerly allergic to back into your diet. Health food stores have a variety of products, such as gluten-free items, for those who are allergic.

YOU DON'T NEED ACYCLOVIR

In 1984, scientists announced the first successful treatment to suppress or prevent recurring attacks of genital herpes in those infected with the fast-spreading, sexually transmitted disease, reported Philip M. Boffey in *The New York Times*. The then-experimental treatment, which involved daily oral doses of the drug Acyclovir, was said to end the physical and emotional trauma experienced by the most severely affected herpes victims. And the scientists speculated that the treatments might reduce the likelihood that herpes victims would spread the disease to their sexual partners, although the researchers admitted that that had not been proved.[1]

"This is not a cure—we are far from a cure," Stephen E. Straus, M.D., head of the medical virology section at the National Institute of Allergy and Infectious Diseases in Washington, D.C., was quoted as saying.

Straus explained that after a flare-up, the herpes virus retreats into the nerve roots and reemerges periodically. The typical patient suffers three or four such flare-ups annually, but those most severely afflicted may experience 12 to 16 recurrences a year. According to Straus, these episodes often destroy social and marital relations, disrupt job performance and result in depression in many people.

Several studies using the drug found that when daily drug treatments stopped, the symptoms reappeared, indicating that the drug had not eradicated the virus or "cured" the patient but merely suppressed the recurrence of symptoms.

Acyclovir (pronounced ay-SYE-kloe-veer) is a medication used to treat infections caused by viruses. It is also known as "Aciclovir" and "Acycloguanosine," and its brand name in the United States and Canada is Zovirax. It is available in capsules and tablets and as an ointment with a doctor's prescription.

Acyclovir ointment is used on the skin and mucous membranes to treat the symptoms of herpes simplex virus infections of the skin, mucous membranes and genitals, according to *The Complete Drug Reference*. However, before using this medication, tell your doctor if you have had any unusual allergic reactions to it in the past. Also tell your doctor or pharmacist if you are allergic to any preservatives or dyes. Topical Acyclovir has not been studied in pregnant women, and, so far, it has not been determined whether topical Acyclovir passes into breast milk. In addition, there is no specific information about the use of topical Acyclovir in the elderly.[2]

"You may experience mild pain, burning or stinging after applying the ointment to open sores," reported *The New Consumer Drug Digest*. "This may be due to direct irritation (touch); try to rub the ointment in gently. Contact your doctor if these symptoms are severe. If a rash and itching occur, contact your doctor immediately; these may be symptoms of an allergic reaction."[3]

Acyclovir ointment does not prevent the spread of infection or the recurrence of sores. So don't use the medication as a preventive because this may lead to the development of strains of the virus that are resistant to Acyclovir. And do not use more of the ointment or use it more often or for longer than your doctor tells you. Do not apply Acyclovir ointment to your eyes unless your doctor directs you to do so. Also, use rubber gloves when applying the ointment to prevent spreading the infection.

Common side effects when using Acyclovir are lightheadedness, headache and skin rash, according to Edward Edelson in *The ABCs of Prescription Drugs*. Less common side effects include bloody urine, breathing difficulties, confusion, hallucinations, nausea, loss of appetite, trembling, vomiting and excessive sweating.[4]

The risk of kidney damage is increased when Acyclovir is taken with other drugs that affect kidney function, including many antibiotics. Overdoses may cause convulsion, hallucinations or kidney shutdown. Older people may experience light-headedness, hallucinations and other adverse mental effects. Large doses of Acyclovir have also interferred with implantation of the fetus in some animal tests.

In its ads for Zovirax in medical journals, Burroughs Wellcome Co. needed a full page of small type to explain some of the drug's possible side effects.[5] For example, the short-term administration of the medication for herpes simplex caused nausea and/or vomiting in 8 of 298 patient treatments (2.7 percent) and headache in 2 of 298 patients (0.6 percent). Less frequent complaints during 298 patient treatments included diarrhea, dizziness, anorexia, fatigue, edema, skin rash, leg pain, inguinal adenopathy (swelling in the groin), medication taste and sore throat.

During long-term administration of the drug, twice daily for one year, in 586 patients, researchers reported these side effects: nausea (4.8 percent), diarrhea (2.4 percent), headache (1.9 percent) and rash (1.7 percent). Side effects for 589 control patients receiving intermittent treatment of recurrences with Zovirax for one year included: diarrhea (2.7 percent), nausea (2.4 percent), headache (2.2 percent) and rash (1.5 percent).

The most frequent adverse reactions reported during three clinical trials of treatment of herpes zoster (shingles) in 323 patients were malaise (11.5 percent), nausea (8.0 percent), headache (5.9 percent), vomiting (2.5 percent), and diarrhea (1.5 percent) and constipation (0.9 percent).

In using the medication for chicken pox, researchers found that 3.2 percent complained of diarrhea, 0.6 percent of abdominal pain, 0.6 percent of vomiting and 0.4 percent of flatulence. Zovirax has caused decreased production of sperm at high injected doses in some animals and mutations in some studies of high concentrations of the drug.

MEET MELISSA

Melissa officinalis L., a member of the Lamiaceae family, is a universal folk remedy with numerous applications. It is also known as lemon balm, sweet balm, honey plant, balm mint, blue balm, common balm, garden balm and many others. It belongs to the mint family.

Lemon balm, which has the square stem that characterizes the mint family, grows from one to two feet high and has ovate, toothed leaves, reported Gaea and Shandor Weiss in *Growing and Using Healing Herbs*. Its white or yellowish flowers appear in small bunches in midsummer. The plant prefers shady places and rich, moist soil. If you plant a lemon balm seed, it will germinate in three to four weeks. Gardeners suggest that you sow seed indoors in late spring and then plant the seedlings outside when they are about four inches tall. The plant can also be grown from root divisions taken in the early spring. In the autumn, the top growth dies back, and the plant can be mulched with compost or leaf mold to enrich the growing environment and provide some winter protection. Although the plant will spread, it does more slowly than most of the other mints.[1]

Melissa, which is rich in such essential oils as peppermint and thyme, originated in the Near East and quickly found its way to Europe and across the Alps, according to Mannifried Pahlow in *Healing Plants*. In his treatise on the management of the royal estates (*Capitulare de villis*), Charlemagne directed, about A.D. 810, that his subjects plant Melissa throughout his domain. Today it continues to grow in many gardens as a medicinal plant and for culinary use.[2]

The Greeks named the herb Melissa, or honeybee, because

its fragrant flowers were so attractive to bees. *Officinalis* is a botanist's term indicating the herb's common use and availability.[3]

One of the sacred herbs in the Temple of Diana, Melissa was prescribed by the ancients for longevity, memory, fertility and an aid to beekeepers, who were encouraged to rub the herb on their beehives. Melissa has long been an ingredient in several commercial European rheumatism ointments as well as in such liqueurs as Chartreuse, Benedictine and the once famous Carmelite Water.[4]

Melissa was held in high esteem in early medicine and was widely used by the Arabs in Spain, according to Francesco Bianchini and Francesco Corbetta in *The Complete Book of Health Plants*. Avicenna, the great Arab physician and philosopher of the 11th century, believed that "it causeth the mind and heart to become merry." It was also known in early cookery, especially as an ingredient in the aromatic liqueurs distilled in Italian monasteries. Melissa is used as a flavoring for certain cheeses in parts of Switzerland, and it is widely used in domestic cookery in salads, omelettes and summer drinks, such as May wine. Culpepper, in his 17th-century herbal, recommends a syrup made of Melissa and sugar to " 'be kept in every gentlewoman's house to relieve the weak stomachs and sick bodies of their poor and sickly neighbors.' "[5]

Melissa was highly esteemed by Paracelsus, who believed it would completely revivify a man, according to Mrs. M. Grieve in *A Modern Herbal*. She quoted the *London Dispensary* (1696): " 'An essence of Balm, given in Canary wine, every morning will renew youth, strengthen the brain, relieve languishing nature and prevent baldness.' "[6]

Hildegarde von Bingen, the Abbess of Rupertsberg, was perhaps the chief herbalist of the 12th century. In her natural science work, *Physica*, she includes Melissa, although under the name *binsung*. In addition to its use against rheumatism, Hildegarde also reported: "And like salt, when added in quantities, it tempers all foodstuff; it feels bad, when too much or too little of it is added; when added in moderate quantities, this Roman preparation gives a good taste and spices meat and fish and foodstuff and mash. When eaten in that manner, it warms the stomach and provides an excellent digestion."[7]

According to historians, the first mention of Melissa appeared around 300 B.C. in *Historia Plantarum*, compiled by Theophrastus of Ephesus, who was a pupil of Aristotle. Noting that bees were attracted to the herb, Theophrastus named it Melissophyllon (bee-balm), according to R. H. Woelbling and K. Leonhardt in *Phytomedicine* in 1994.[8]

Between about 50 and 80 A.D., Plinus Secundus, a Roman, recommended Melissa for therapeutic use in his *Materia Medica*, since it had been used externally to treat insect bites and internally for the treatment of abdominal colic and uterine spasms. During the Middle Ages, the medical school at Salerno praised the sedative qualities of Melissa, and this usage persists to this day.

Melissa has been used medicinally for more than 20 centuries, usually as a sedative, spasmolytic or for its antibacterial properties, according to Varro E. Tyler, Ph.D., Sc.D., in *Herbs of Choice: The Therapeutic Use of Phytomedicinals*. These effects are attributed primarily to a volatile oil, which is contained in quality plant material in concentrations of at least 0.05 percent. Some of the chief constituents of the oil include citronellal, citral A, citral B and many other mono- and sesquiterpenes. The German Commission E has found Melissa to be a safe and effective calmative and carminative.

"It was first demonstrated in 1978 that an aqueous extract of Melissa, containing a variety of polyphenolic substances, including oxidation products of caffeic acid and its derivatives, demonstrated antiviral activity," said Tyler. "The caffeic acid oxidation product is said to inhibit not only herpes simplex type 1 virus, which causes cold sores, but also the herpes simplex type 2, which causes genital herpes."[9]

A pharmaceutical product for external use, now available as a Melissa ointment concentrated 70:1, is sold in both Europe and the United States. It contains a unique concentrated extract of Melissa which is only produced by the Lomapharm Company of Germany. Application of the ointment two to four times daily is said to shorten the healing time of the lesions associated with herpes and to decrease their recurrence rate.

Various researchers have determined that the main active constituents in Melissa are an essential oil containing monoterpenoid aldehydes—geranial (Alpha Citral), neral (Beta Citral) and citronellal—flavonoids, including glycosides of luteolin and quercetin; monoterpene and phenyl propanoid glycosides; hydroxycinnamic derivatives including caffeic and chlorogenic acids and rosmarinic acid.

MELISSA TO THE RESCUE

The initial investigations of the antiviral activity of water extracts of *Melissa officinalis* in 1964 demonstrated their ability to inhibit the spread of various types of virus, including vaccinia and herpes simplex. Studies by other researchers over the next ten years or so corroborated these first findings.

Later, within the framework of an extensive project seeking naturally occurring antiviral compounds, another group of researchers undertook elaborate studies with aqueous extracts from 178 species of medicinal plants belonging to 69 botanical families. Their purpose was to determine the antiviral properties of these plants against herpes, influenza, vaccinia and polio viruses. Extracts from 75 of the 178 species were found to produce inhibitory activities against one or more of the viruses. The study provided evidence that the extracts from the Laminacea species displayed marked antiviral activity and low cytotoxicity. Following further tests, preference was given to *Melissa officinalis*, a member of the Laminacea family, since its various properties showed significant antiviral potency with no toxic side effects. With this information, a German pharmaceutical company, in consultations with May and Willuhn in 1979 and 1980, developed a process whereby the main constituents of Melissa could be extracted.[1]

Further investigations confirmed that the antiviral activity of the extract from *Melissa officinalis* is due to its glucosidically bound phenolcarbonic acids and their polymers.

Clinical studies in 1982 and 1989 confirmed the efficacy of the German-made Melissa 70:1 extract cream for herpes simplex infections, and the cream has been a registered medicine by Lomapharm in Germany since 1983. Further research led to the development of a 2 percent solution of the Melissa extract for the treatment of the varicella-zoster viral infection.

"The Melissa leaves, used for the manufacture of the extract, must conform to the specifications set forth in the current edition of DAB (German Pharmacopoeia)," wrote R. H. Woelbling and K. Leonhardt in *Phytomedicine* in 1994. "The standardization of the extract in terms of the antiviral potency is ensured by the use of specially selected drugs, strict implementation of the prescribed manufacturing process, and the relevant chromatographic analyses and virological tests."[2]

As reported earlier, the identity and chemical composition of the Melissa leaves are confirmed by the chromatographic HPLC-fingerprint analysis, using caffeic acid, chlorogenic acid and rosmarinic acid. The antiviral potency of the Melissa leaves is determined by appropriate virological tests. Researchers use a modified method of the generally known *in vitro* plaque inhibition test, also used for the exploration of new antiviral agents.

CLINICAL STUDIES

Writing in *Phytomedicine* in 1994, R. H. Woelbling and K. Leonhardt described clinical studies in Germany at three dermatological clinics and a private clinic using Melissa to treat the herpes simplex virus. The studies involved 115 patients, including 45 males and 70 females. Those accepted for the studies were patients with a herpes simplex infection of the skin or transitional mucosa whose clinical symptoms had lasted for not more than 72 hours prior to entering the study. Excluded from the study group were those with any known hypersensitivity to the ingredients in the Melissa cream or other treatments that had been prescribed for a viral infection. Each patient received one tube of the test preparation which contained 5 grams of the Melissa 70:1 cream.

During each study, the volunteers were advised to apply the cream at home five times daily until healing of the lesion was complete. The study lasted for 14 days. Researchers documented the clinical symptoms at the beginning of the study and subsequently on days 4, 6 and 8 of the treatment. The following data were recorded for later examination: date of the first examination, site of the lesion, the onset of the clinical symptoms (in hours), healing of the vesicular eruption and side-effects, if any.

The researchers determined that healing of the lesions was complete in 96 percent of the patients until day 8 of the treatment and 60 percent and 87 percent on days 4 and 6, respectively.

"Three of the 115 patients treated with the test preparation complained of a sensation of burning and paresthesia (prickling)," reported Woelbling and Leonhardt. "Any conclusive correlation between these side effects and the application of the test preparation being examined could not be established, since such symptoms are also characteristic of the herpes simplex infection itself. It can be inferred from the results of the study that the application of the Melissa extract incorporated in a cream base brought about a speedy healing of the herpetic lesions. Natural recovery from herpetic infection of the skin or transitional mucosa usually occurs within 10 to 14 days."[1]

A randomized placebo-controlled, double-blind study was carried out at two German dermatological centers. Case reports of the 116 outpatients were evaluated prior to the study. The placebo group was composed of 44 females and 14 males, compared with 41 females and 17 males in the Melissa group. Average age of the patients in the placebo group was 33.2 ± 14.8 years, compared with 40.3 ± 14.8 years in the Melissa group. In the Berlin study, three children were in the placebo group, ages 4, 5 and 6.

During the study, the volunteers were given either the Melissa cream containing 5 grams of the extract or a placebo containing 5 grams of cream without the Melissa extract. The patients were told to apply the Melissa cream or the placebo two to four times daily on the affected areas of the skin for 5 to 10 days. As with the previous trials, volunteers had a herpes simplex infection of the skin or transitional mucosa, with clinical symptoms lasting not more than 72 hours prior to admission to the study.

Case histories were obtained from each patient during the initial consultation, and the following data were evaluated:

- Date of first examination.
- Site of the lesion.
- Prodromal sensations (pain, burning, itching, prickling and so on).
- The onset of the prodromal sensations (in hours).
- The appearance of the symptoms on the skin (in hours).

- Beginning of the treatment (date).
- Former treatment (no, yes, which?).

Clinical symptoms were categorized as follows:

- Rubor (none, slight, moderate, severe).
- Swelling (none, slight, moderate, severe).
- Vesicles (none, few and superficial, many, many and deep).
- Scabs (none, few, many, falling off).
- Pain (none, slight, severe, extremely severe).
- Healing (complete, partial, no).

The duration of the prodromal signs was virtually the same in both groups: 21.2 ± 19.0 hours in the Melissa group and 21.3 ± 19.0 hours in the placebo group. The clinical symptoms in the placebo group appeared 14.0 ± 12.6 hours before the treatment, compared with 18.5 ± 17.5 hours in the Melissa group. In other words, a statistically significant difference did not exist. In the placebo group, 40 patients did not have any former treatment and 18 patients had undergone a treatment before the study; in the Melissa group, the corresponding figures were 25 and 13, respectively. Lesions on the lips represented the highest incidence with 34 and 33 cases, respectively, in the two trial groups. Genital herpes was diagnosed in four and six patients, respectively, in the two groups.

On the fifth and final day of the trial, the researchers found no symptoms in 24 patients using the Melissa cream, as contrasted with 15 patients using the placebo. On the second day, the researchers reported that the decline of the symptoms in the Melissa group was statistically more significant than in the placebo group. Concerning symptoms such as vesication, scabbing, erosion and pain, there was no significant difference in the two trial groups under the conditions of the study design. However, it was pointed out that scabbing in the Melissa group was less than in those using the placebo, suggesting reduced damage of the cells in the Melissa group.

In the overall assessment during the course of healing—global evaluation by the physician and the patient—there was a conclusive difference between the Melissa and the placebo groups, indicating that the healing in the Melissa group was statistically significant.

In a study involving the use of Melissa against cold sores, 67 patients were evaluated. Thirty-three volunteers were assigned to the Melissa group and 34 to the placebo group. Judged by the decline of lesions, the healing in the patients of the Melissa group was faster than in those of the placebo group. The researchers added that even for those patients who had to undergo a therapeutic treatment within six hours after the initial appearance of the symptoms, the decline of the area of the lesion until the termination of the treatment was still significantly faster in the Melissa group when compared with the placebo group.

Concerning side effects, the researchers said that there was no statistical difference in the two trial groups. In the placebo group, irritation developed in two patients and two patients also complained of a sense of burning. In the Melissa group, one patient complained of irritation at the time of the second followup examination. Three volunteers withdrew from the study, including two from the Melissa group and one from the placebo group. In one of the patients using the Melissa cream, there was an exacerbation of symptoms. The second patient gave no reason for not continuing the study.

"In the present study," the researchers continued, "the Melissa cream revealed itself as being significantly and highly superior to the placebo during the very critical initial stage of the treatment. Also, the decline of swelling on the second day of the treatment with Melissa was significantly more pronounced than with the placebo. In the global assessment of efficacy, the Melissa cream was judged as conclusively superior to the placebo by both physician and patient."

The researchers added that the results of this study are

more remarkable in that the studies carried out in the United States with idoxuridine, Acyclovir and 5-ara-AMP had revealed no benefits distinguished from the placebo, except that in two subgroups the drug proved statistically superior to placebo with regard to the clinical symptoms. Only one clinical study in the United Kingdom demonstrated that Acyclovir was superior to the placebo. It is worth noting that in a 1984 study the decline of virus titre in the vascular fluid due to treatment with 10 percent Acyclovir was not significantly different from that due to the placebo. The results of the study with Melissa extract, in contrast with the just-named studies, provide the convincing argument that it is of value in the treatment of herpes simplex diseases. Concerning side effects, no allergic contract reactions were noticed.

The researchers noted that, to be effective, treatment with Melissa must be started in the early stages of the infection. An additional merit of the Melissa extract in topical use is that it does not induce any viral resistance.

It is recommended that people with herpes take the Melissa cream with them while traveling, especially if they will be exposed to high levels of ultraviolet radiation at a beach, on the water or in the mountains. Depending on the severity of the infection, treatment should continue for four to eight days. To avoid spreading the virus, apply the cream to areas surrounding the lesions. Physicians also suggest that the cream be applied for several days after relief of symptoms.[2]

CASE HISTORIES

The following five case histories, collected at random during 1994, illustrate the effectiveness of the Melissa extract cream in treating various types of herpes infections.

Case 1: K. H., a 61-year-old woman

She had a history of recurring *Herpes labialis*, an infection on the lip. She consulted her doctor because of the classical prodromal signs and the fresh blisters on the reddened background. The skin on the lower lip was also affected. She was advised to use the Melissa cream three times daily. After two days of treatment with the cream, the blisters had subsided and only a slight redness of the skin could be detected.

Case 2: F. B., a 64-year-old woman

This patient also suffered from a recurring herpes simplex infection of the lower lip. She had noticed the initial lesion about 24 hours earlier, which led to a painful blister and lesions at the edge of the lip. After seven days of treatment with the Melissa cream, the lesions were completely healed.

Case 3: M. D., a 46-year-old man

He was hospitalized with *Psoriasis vulgaris*, which had been intensively treated with ultraviolet-B (UV-B) irradiation. The radiation resulted in a herpes solaris blister on his upper lip. Since the patient was in the hospital, the Melissa cream was administered five hours after the onset of the symptoms. (To ensure rapid healing, it is important to apply the cream as soon as possible after the onset of prodromal signs.) After two days of treatment, the blister formation had already begun to subside.

Case 4: C. K., a 15-year-old girl

This patient was diagnosed with a herpes blister formation just below the nose. The Melissa cream was applied 36 hours after the onset of the illness. A cluster of lesions was about 0.6 centimeter in size. After seven days of Melissa treatment, there was considerable healing under a slight formation of crusts. Some acne lesions were also detected.

Case 5: B. R., a 55-year-old man

This patient had also been admitted to the hospital with *Psoriasis vulgaris*. After a strong dose of UV-B, a large area with herpes glutealis on the right side was detected. This reddened area was about 2.5 centimeters in diameter. The partly cloudy blisters appeared about 48 hours after the initial finding.

After four days with a Melissa treatment, the blisters were completely dried up. Some slight crusts were formed and a remaining erythema could be seen. Even this vast herpes infection was resolved after nine days of treatment. Only a slight remaining erosion near the crusts could be detected.

THE FUTURE OF PHYTOTHERAPY

The results with Melissa in curbing herpes simplex outbreaks give a clear picture regarding the phytotherapy of the future, according to Wolf G. Dorner. The use of medicinal plants in modern therapy will no longer be based on what is known presently, that is, experience. Cooperation among chemists, biologists, bacteriologists, pharmacists and medical professionals will increasingly lead to a phytotherapy that is more and more based on scientific facts. This will remove the criticism that therapy with medicinal plants is a nonscientific approach, because the effects cannot be demonstrated. Therefore, the phytotherapy of the future will not play second fiddle to chemotherapy; it will be a targeted effort.

Many phytopharmaceutical agents exhibit a weak effect. Therefore, they are well suited to fight diseases that must be treated over a long period of time. These agents have the advantage of producing a therapeutic effect only after an initial period. However, this does not make them second-class agents. Just the opposite is true.

"An accurate knowledge will exist regarding the effect of a preparation (i.e., what component has what effect)," said Dorner. "Furthermore, phytopharmaceutical agents will exhibit the advantage that the side effects are kept to a minimum, when they are properly manufactured and used according to the directions. They will distinctly broaden the therapeutic spectrum and thus help to improve the supply to the patient. The requirements placed on modern preparations are, therefore, met."[1]

References

Foreword

1. Bill Gottlieb, ed., *New Choices in Natural Healing* (Emmaus, Pa.: Rodale Press, Inc., 1995), pp. 247, 323.
2. Varro E. Tyler, Ph.D., "Plant Drugs in the 21st Century" *Economic Botany* 40, no. 3 (1986): 279–88.

Introduction

1. Robert M. Giller, M.D., and Kathy Matthews, "Herpes," in *Natural Prescriptions* (New York: Carol Southern Books, 1994), p. 182.
2. Alma E. Guinness, *ABC's of the Human Body* (Pleasantville, N.Y.: The Reader's Digest Association, 1987), p. 278.
3. Carol Potera, "The Herpes Double Standard," *Longevity* (September 1995), p. 58.
4. Jeffrey R. M. Kunz, editor-in-chief, *The American Medical Association Family Medical Guide* (New York: Random House, 1982), pp. 316, 451.
5. Ann Hill, et al., "Herpes Simplex Virus Turns Off the TAP to Evade Host Immunity," *Nature* 375 (1995): 411–15.
6. Richard A. Knox, "New Clues to Fatigue Syndrome: Brain Inflamma-

tion, Viral Infection Found in Most Patients Studied," (*Sacramento Bee* 15 January 1992.)

7. Joseph Melnick and Arni Schattner, "Viruses and Atherosclerosis," *Israel Journal of Medical Sciences* 28 (1992): 463–64.

Learning More About Your Skin

1. Jeffrey R. M. Kunz, M.D., editor-in-chief, *The American Medical Association Family Medical Guide* (New York: Random House, 1982), pp. 250–51.
2. Cathey Pinckney and Edward R. Pinckney, M.D., *Do-It-Yourself Medical Testing* (New York: Facts On File, 1989), pp. 74ff.

How Herpes Enters a Cell

1. Natalie Angier, "Researchers Determine How Herpes Enters the Cell," *The New York Times* (15 June 1990), p. A12.

Cold Sores and Fever Blisters

1. Genell J. Subak-Sharpe, ed. *The Physicians' Manual for Patients* (New York: Times Books, 1984), p. 365.
2. Eberhard Kronhausen, Ed.D., et al., *Formula for Life* (New York: William Morrow & Co., Inc., 1989), p. 187.
3. Robert M. Ossoff, D.M.D., M.D., and Michael J. Koriwchak, M.D., "Lip Sores," *Medical and Health Annual* (Chicago: Encyclopaedia Britannica, Inc., 1992), p. 458.

Genital Herpes

1. Bernadine Healy, M.D., *A New Prescription for Women's Health* (New York: Viking, 1995), p. 154.
2. Kenneth Seaton, "Hygiene and the Incidence of AIDS?" *High Tech Hygiene* (October 1991), handout leaflet.
3. Rick A. Barbarash, Pharm.D., et al., "Psychosocial Stress and Adjustment Among Women with Chronic Recurrent Genital Herpes" *Journal of the Advancement of Medicine* 7, no. 2 (Summer 1994): 77–86.

The Chicken Pox Connection

1. Jeffrey R. M. Kunz, M.D., editor-in-chief, *The American Medical Association Family Guide* (New York: Random House, 1982), p. 700.
2. Howard R. Lewis and Martha E. Lewis, *The People's Medical Manual* (Garden City, N.Y.: Doubleday & Co., Inc., 1986), p. 144.
3. Genell J. Subak-Sharpe, ed., *The Physicians' Manual for Patients* (New York: Times Books, 1984), p. 370.

Where Shingles Fits In

1. Jeffrey R. M. Kunz, M.D., editor-in-chief, *The American Medical Association Family Medical Guide* (New York: Random House, 1982), pp. 562–63.
2. Howard R. Lewis and Martha E. Lewis, *The People's Medical Manual* (Garden City, N.Y.: Doubleday & Co., Inc., 1986), p. 479.
3. Michael Oxman, M.D., "Shingles," *The Institute for Research on Aging Newsletter* 9, no. 7. (March 1989):3.

What Herpes Tests Are Available

1. David S. Sobel, M.D., and Tom Ferguson, M.D., *The People's Book of Medical Tests* (New York: Summit Books, 1985), pp. 143–44.
2. Marcia Holle, "First Rapid Test for Herpes Now Available," news release from Ruder Finn & Rotman, Inc., New York, 6 December 1985.

Are Allergies Involved?

1. Thomas R. Klosinski, D.C., *The Herpes Handbook* (Greenbrae, Calif.: Alternative Treatment Programs, Inc., 1983), pp. 15ff.

You Don't Need Acyclovir

1. Philip M. Boffey, "Treatment Found to Prevent Flareup of Herpes Symptoms," *The New York Times*, 14 June 1984, 1.
2. *The Complete Drug Reference* (Mount Vernon, N.Y.: Consumer Reports Books, 1991), pp. 24ff.
3. American Society of Hospital Pharmacists, *The New Consumer Drug Digest* (New York: Facts on File, 1985), pp. 187ff.
4. Edward Edelson, *The ABC's of Prescription Drugs* (Garden City, N.Y.: Doubleday & Co., Inc., 1987), p. 254.
5. Ad for Zovirax, Burroughs Wellcome Co., March 1995.

Meet Melissa

1. Gaea and Shandor Weiss, *Growing and Using Healing Herbs* (Emmaus, Pa.: Rodale Press, 1985), pp. 173ff.
2. Mannifried Pahlow, *Healing Plants* (Hauppauge, N.Y.: Barron's Educational Services, Inc., 1992), p. 182
3. Robert Shosteck, *Flowers and Plants: An International Lexicon with Biographical Notes* (New York: Quadrangle/The New York Times Book Co., 1974), p. 14.
4. Michelle Mairesse, *Health Secrets of Medicinal Plants* (New York: Arco, 1981), pp. 11–12.
5. Francesco Bianchini and Francesco Corbetta, *The Complete Book of Health Plants* (New York: Crescent Books, 1975), p. 18.

6. Mrs. M. Grieve, *A Modern Herbal* (New York: Dover Publications, Inc., 1971), pp. 76–77.
7. Wolf G. Dorner, "Melissa—Still Capable of a Surprise or Two," *Pharmazie in unserer Zeit* 14, no. 4 (1985): 3–4.
8. R. H. Woelbling and K. Leonhardt, "Local Therapy of Herpes Simplex with Dried Extract from Melissa Officinalis," *Phytomedicine* 1 (1994): 25–31.
9. Varro E. Tyler, Ph.D., Sc.D., *Herbs of Choice: The Therapeutic Use of Phytomedicinals* (New York: Pharmaceutical Products Press, 1994), p. 165.

Melissa to the Rescue

1. "Monograph for Lomaherpan Creme," Lomapharm, February 1994.
2. R. H. Woelbling and K. Leonhardt, "Local Therapy of Herpes Simplex with Dried Extract from Melissa Officinalis," *Phytomedicine* 1 (1994): 25–31.

Clinical Studies

1. R. H. Woelbling and K. Leonhardt, "Local Therapy of Herpes Simplex with Dried Extract from Melissa Officinalis," *Phytomedicine* 1 (1994): 25–31.
2. Brochure from the Lomapharm Company, undated.

The Future of Phytotherapy

1. Wolf G. Dorner, "Melissa: Still Capable of a Surprise of Two," *Pharmazie in unserer Zeit* 14, no. 4 (1985): 23.